Optimal Functioning
A Positive Psychology Handbook

Revised Edition

Jessica D. Colman, MAPP

Foreword by Daniel S. Bowling, III

Edited by Brighid Desmond
and Margaret Ulrich

Abstract

The Optimal Functioning handbook consists of a series of concise chapters on topics relating to well-being, happiness, and personal success. It is written for the use of individuals, coaches, educators, and other professionals interested in applying positive psychology to enhance well-being. The handbook provides straightforward summaries of key positive psychology research findings, interventions, themes, and areas of study. It also includes actionable suggestions for applying the empirical findings in one's life. The handbook was written with the intention of increasing the availability of positive psychology's knowledge and tools for the general population, so that they can be applied to help individuals, organizations, and societies flourish.

"I did not choose positive psychology. It called me."
-Martin Seligman

Table of Contents

Foreword by Daniel S. Bowling, III

Introduction to Positive Psychology

Well-being Theory

Character Strengths and Values in Action (VIA)

Positive Emotions, Negative Emotions, and "Negativity Bias"

Flow

Goal-Setting

Motivation

Self-Regulation

Altruism and Giving

Gratitude

Savoring

Hope

Active Constructive Responding

Excess Choice

Coaching

Appreciative Inquiry

Resilience

Conclusion

Acknowledgments

References

I teach at the University of Pennsylvania in a graduate program offering a master's degree in "Positive Psychology." Despite its somewhat off-putting name, with a faint whiff of self-help and happy talk, it is an extraordinarily rigorous program, a scientific study of the "good life" and all that makes life worth living. It is supervised - quite actively - by Dr. Martin E.P. Seligman, a no-nonsense Ivy League academic who might be the greatest psychologist of our generation, and Dr. James Pawelski, a philosopher of the first rate and a leading authority on the 19th Century psychologist William James.

Positive psychology is psychology, and as such is science, subject to the same methods of empirical analysis as all the sciences. To broadly summarize the main premise of the discipline, it is an assertion that psychological health is more than the absence of disease, it is about human flourishing. It challenges scientists and practitioners to place as much time and energy on helping humans live the best life they can - a notion not unfamiliar to those who study Aristotle - as they do avoiding illness. Critically, positive psychology does not attempt to ignore problems or replace traditional psychology, but aims to complement current areas of knowledge. Those who focus in this area, and our ranks are growing, believe the positive elements of life are just as important as the negative, and deserve their own academic and scientific exploration.

The program attracts interesting, diverse people. Like Jessica Colman, a graduate of the University of California - San Diego. A quiet, striking young lady, modest and unassuming, she asked me last spring to be the advisor on her master's thesis paper, or "capstone." I expected something of high quality from Jessica, given her outstanding performance as a student, but found much, much more—possibly the most practical guide yet written for persons seeking to understand and apply the major tenets of positive psychology.

That is the handbook you have before you: Optimal Functioning: A Positive Psychology Handbook. It is a compact yet comprehensive guide that belongs on the bookshelf and briefcase - or digital library - of anyone interested in this topic. I keep a well-marked copy with me much of the time, and refer to it often when teaching, working with coaching clients, writing, or in need of an attitudinal tune-up myself.

The handbook covers 16 of the most popular topics for researchers and practitioners of positive psychology, topics such as motivation, positive emotion, and character strengths and virtues. Each is the subject of its own chapter and is broken down into two parts. Take the chapter on "Hope," for example. First, with economy of expression, Colman reviews the empirical studies on hope and what science has to tell us about why it is important to psychological health. Then, she offers concrete suggestions—yes, she calls them "tips"—for developing hope and applying it in one's life or with clients. It is partly an academic overview, partly a "how to" manual—and useful for both purposes. Read it for either.

This is a fast read, but a deep one. Refer to it often. Jump between chapters. Send it to a friend or favorite client. Find meaning in its pages, and maybe help someone in the process. Even yourself.

The emerging world of positive psychology and those who labor in the field need a handbook like this. And we owe thanks to Jessica Colman for writing it.

Daniel S. Bowling, III   Duke Law School   Thanksgiving, 2010

Introduction to Positive Psychology

In the late 1990s, Martin Seligman named the field of positive psychology and made its principles the theme of his term as president of the American Psychological Association (Peterson, 2006). He and his colleagues brought attention to the fact that the field of psychology had almost exclusively focused on pathology, or repairing damage within a disease model of functioning. As a result, it had very little knowledge of the fulfilled individual, the thriving community, or other positive features that make life worth living (Seligman, & Csikszentmihalyi, 2000).

Positive psychology attempts to balance the field of psychology and make it more complete by shifting the focus from repairing the worst things in life to enhancing the positive aspects. This can improve quality of life and prevent the pathologies that arise when life is empty and meaningless. The field of positive psychology has grown and established itself as the scientific study of the factors that allow individuals, communities, and societies to flourish. It studies the "good life" by focusing on positive individual traits, positive subjective experiences, and positive institutions (Seligman, & Csikszentmihalyi, 2000).

Though the field is new, the subject, and even the name, are not. Positive psychologists study the same questions concerning the "good life" as those posed by great thinkers and philosophers such as Confucius and Aristotle, and religious figures such as Buddha and Mohammed. Contemporary positive psychology has synthesized what were previously isolated lines of theory and research, and argues that the aspects of life that make it worth living deserve their own field of inquiry within psychology (Peterson, 2006). A central goal of positive psychology's research and study is to articulate a vision of the "good life" that is empirically sound, while at the same time reasonable and desirable (Seligman, & Csikszentmihalyi, 2000).

Though in some ways the field of positive psychology is young, it already contains a great deal of knowledge concerning the "good life" and its attainment. This quick reference guide has been created to provide people with simple and straightforward summaries of important concepts, and the means to apply them to enable optimal functioning. It is a tool for sharing and disseminating positive psychology's current knowledge of what constitutes the "good life," and how to achieve it.

<u>Well-being Theory</u>

In December 2003, Martin Seligman published <u>Authentic Happiness</u>, which became many people's initial introduction to the field of positive psychology. At that time, Seligman believed that the topic of positive psychology was happiness, which is operationalized or measured by life satisfaction. Thus, Authentic Happiness Theory described happiness and its elements, which Seligman argued to be positive emotion, engagement, and meaning. The book introduced ideas such as using strength-based approaches in psychology and discussed methods of cultivating positive emotions, virtue, and positive institutions. The publishing of <u>Authentic Happiness</u> was part of a paradigm shift that corresponded with the birth of positive psychology, and sparked much interest and debate. However, it did not stop there for Seligman, who continued to refine his theories and views of the field after <u>Authentic Happiness</u>.

Through his continued investigation, Seligman came to identify a number of problems with Authentic Happiness Theory. One of these problems is that the popular understanding of happiness is largely related to positive emotion, and doesn't adequately take into account engagement and meaning. This is problematic, because some people do not experience large amounts of positive emotion, but their lives may be full of engagement and meaning. "Happiness" wasn't broad enough to describe the "good life" to Seligman's satisfaction. Another problem he grappled with was the fact that life satisfaction, a subjective, self-reported measure, was the only way to measure happiness. Life satisfaction varies greatly depending on the mood people are in when they self-report. In fact, mood can determine more than 70% of the life satisfaction reported (Seligman, 2011). He wrote, "Life satisfaction essentially measures cheerful mood, so it is not entitled to a central place in any theory that aims to be more than a happiology" (Seligman, 2011, p.14). Finally, he felt that positive emotion, engagement, and meaning did not form an exhaustive list of the things that people pursue "for their own sake." That is, there are other things that people will pursue even if they receive no positive emotion, engagement, or meaning from doing so. Seligman felt that his theory should be broad enough to include those other factors.

It was these issues, along with inspiration that came as the field and his experiences evolved, that led Seligman to articulate a new theory he calls Well-being Theory. In April 2011 he published <u>Flourish: A Visionary New Understanding of Happiness and Well-being</u>, which discussed the new theory and many new discoveries within positive psychology since <u>Authentic Happiness</u> was published. In <u>Flourish</u>, Seligman explains that he now believes the topic of positive psychology is well-being rather than happiness. He explains that well-being is a construct while happiness is a "thing." Things can be directly measured, while constructs have several measurable elements (things) that contribute to it, but none of which define it directly. When deciding on the elements of well-being Seligman used three determining criteria: 1) the element contributes to well-being; 2) many people pursue it for its own sake rather than to receive any of the other elements; and 3) it can be defined and measured independently of the other elements.

Using these criteria he decided on the elements of his well-being construct, which ended up being an expanded version of his initial theory of happiness. The new construct contains positive emotion, engagement, and meaning as pillars of well-being, and adds two more -accomplishment and relationships. He added positive accomplishment because he believes that many people are motivated to pursue success, achievement, and mastery regardless of whether it brings them positive emotion, engagement, or meaning. He added relationships because very little that is good in life is solitary. By studying the evolution of the brain and group selection theory, Seligman came to believe that positive relationships are so basic to the success of the species Homo Sapien, that evolution designed our psychological make-up such that the other elements of well-being support the pursuit of positive relationships. He adds that if happiness or life satisfaction was the sole measure of what humans were motivated to pursue, the human race would have died out long ago. Thus, Seligman's new goal of positive psychology is not to merely increase happiness, but to increase the amount of flourishing in individuals' lives and on the planet. This will be facilitated by an increasing ability for science to measure the elements of well-being and study it with rigor.

<u>**Character Strengths and the VIA**</u>

A strengths perspective or orientation assumes that capitalizing on one's best qualities is likely to lead to greater success than would be possible by making a comparable effort to improve areas of weakness (Lopez, and Louis, 2009). This idea is a core tenet of positive psychology, which was founded with the intention to cultivate mental health rather than cure mental illness. Positive psychology has always been concerned with taking people from zero to +10 on the emotional scale, while traditional psychology focused on taking people from -10 to zero. Taking people from zero to +10 requires cultivating that which is working well and building on strengths.

Using and cultivating one's strengths is a highly individualized form of personal growth and development. "A strengths perspective assumes that every individual has resources that can be mobilized toward success in many areas of life and is characterized by efforts to 'label what is right' within people and organizations" (Lopez, and Louis, 2009, p.2). In addition, using strengths, or doing what a person does best, has been shown to lead to high levels of engagement and productivity (Seligman, 2009). Positive psychology has explored this, and found that strengths can also be used to leverage weaknesses at both an individual and group level. Developing and capitalizing on strengths is a crucial aspect of achievement and flourishing, and it is important for each individual to learn how to mobilize their own strengths most effectively. This can be done by measuring one's strengths and intentionally developing them through application.

Early in positive psychology's history, it became clear that in order to help people evolve toward their highest potential we first had to define concepts such as "strength" and "highest potential," so that they could be assessed and measured (Seligman, 2002). However, topics such as strengths, virtue, and character had been largely ignored in twentieth century academia. Many scholars believed that good character could be cultivated, but they needed conceptual and empirical tools with which to create and evaluate interventions (Peterson, & Seligman, 2004). It is not possible to scientifically intervene to improve character without knowing exactly what you're trying to improve. Thus, a classification of the sanities, or a taxonomy of character was necessary in order to use strengths of character in a scientific pursuit of the "good life." This classification would become the backbone of positive psychology, and positive psychology's answer to the Diagnostic and Statistical Manual of Mental Disorder (DSM) (Seligman, 2002). It would also help legitimize the study of character and virtue in twenty-first century academia.

Martin Seligman recruited Christopher Peterson to lead this initiative. At the time Peterson was a distinguished scientist, author of the leading textbook on personality, a world authority on hope and optimism, and director of the University of Michigan's clinical psychology program (Seligman, 2002). A nonprofit organization called the Values in Action (VIA) Institute was founded with the purpose of developing a scientific knowledge base of human strengths. The first task the Values in Action team took on was to read the fundamental writings and texts of all major religious and philosophical traditions. This included Aristotle, Plato, Aquinas, Augustine, the Old Testament, the Talmud, Confucius, Buddha, Lao-Tze, the Koran, Benjamin Franklin, the Upanishads, the samurai code Bushido, and more – approximately two hundred texts in all. They catalogued that which each tradition claimed were the virtues, and then looked for overarching themes. Their hope was to discover a list of virtues that are ubiquitous across cultures. They found that almost every one of the traditions, spanning the globe and three thousand years, valued and endorsed six common virtues (Seligman, 2002):

Wisdom and knowledge
Courage
Love and humanity
Justice

Temperance
Spirituality and transcendence

The details and methods of achieving these virtues differ across cultures and texts, but there were real and remarkable commonalities (Seligman, 2002). Each virtue can be achieved in a number of ways, and this needed to be further explored in order to measure the virtues and eventually focus on building them. This is where character strengths fit in. According to VIA scholars, character strengths are distinguishable routes to displaying the virtues (Peterson, & Seligman, 2004). For example, the virtue of wisdom can be exhibited through character strengths such as curiosity, love of learning, perspective, open-mindedness, and creativity.

Thus, a classification of 24 character strengths was created, each character strength displaying one of the six categories of virtue. The creators of this VIA classification see it as a starting point, which is currently neither exclusive nor exhaustive, but could be with further research (Peterson, & Seligman, 2004). They had ten specific criteria that the strengths of character had to meet to be included in the classification, such as it needed to be ubiquitously valued across cultures, it must be distinct from other traits in the classification, and it must contribute to various fulfillments of the "good life."

The 24 VIA Character Strengths (Peterson, & Seligman, 2004)

Strengths of Wisdom and Knowledge:

- Creativity
- Curiosity
- Open-Mindedness
- Love of Learning
- Perspective

Strengths of Courage:

- Bravery

- Persistence

- Integrity

- Vitality

Strengths of Humanity:

- Love

- Kindness

- Social Intelligence

Strengths of Justice:

- Citizenship

- Fairness

- Leadership

Strengths of Temperance:

- Forgiveness and Mercy

- Humility and Modesty

- Prudence

- Self-Regulation

Strengths of Transcendence:

- Appreciation of Beauty and Excellence

- Gratitude

- Hope

- Humor

- Spirituality

<u>Tips for Using Strengths-Based Approaches to Individual Development</u>

Start with a Strengths Assessment: It is now possible to measure strengths and other positive personal variables such as hope, engagement, and subjective well-being. The Values in Action (VIA) Survey and the Clifton StrengthsFinder are excellent starting points.

Set Goals Based on Your Strengths: Strengths are cultivated through deliberate application. Create an orientation toward the future that searches for ways to utilize and develop your strengths.

Use Strengths in Novel Ways: Seek out novel experiences and new opportunities to apply your strengths. A good exercise is to attempt to use your strengths in a new way every day.

Use Strengths to Manage Weaknesses: When you have to do something you're not good at or don't like doing, find a way to use your strengths to get it done. In groups, networking and leveraging strengths, or effectively utilizing each group-member's set of strengths for the best of the group, can lead to the highest achievement.

Keep an Eye Out for Strengths in Yourself and Others: "Strengths develop best in response to other human beings" (Lopez, and Louis, 2009, p.4). Make a habit of noticing and identifying strengths in yourself and others. In groups, this can begin a cycle of providing affirmative feedback as people notice the strengths of others and assist in their cultivation. Research has shown that when leaders focus on and invest in the strengths of their employees, the odds of each employee being engaged at work go up eightfold (Rath, & Conchie, 2008).

<u>Positive Emotions, Negative Emotions, and "Negativity Bias"</u>

For many years scientists have understood that negative emotions evolved because they produced behaviors that were adaptive to our human or pre-human ancestors. Negative emotions produce urges to act in particular ways, or produce specific action tendencies (Fredrickson, 2009). Anger produces the urge to attack, fear produces the urge to flee, disgust produces the urge to expel, etc. Thus, negative emotions are important because they are linked to behaviors that helped our ancestors survive the infinite number of life-and-death situations they encountered over the centuries. Negative emotions not only produce behaviors, but also prepare the body to undertake those behaviors. Besides producing the urge to flee, looming danger also mobilizes the cardiovascular and adrenal systems to give muscles more oxygen and energy, preparing the body to run. Emotions infuse an individual's entire being, from their thoughts and actions to their physiological state, and do so in adaptive ways.

Scientists have had a much more difficult time explaining the purpose of positive emotions, or how and why they have evolved as part of our emotional repertoire. Professor Barbara Fredrickson's groundbreaking research has provided insight into this puzzle. She contends that negative emotions narrow people's view of possible actions to those that will help them survive threats. Her "broaden-and-build" theory of positive emotions holds that positive emotions broaden people's view of possible actions, opening their awareness to a wider range of thoughts and actions than is typical (Fredrickson, 2009). This broadened mindset sparked by positive emotions was valuable to our ancestors because over time the expanded awareness built their resources, leading to the development of assets, abilities, and useful traits. The open mindsets that positive emotions produce lead to exploration and experiential learning, through which people gain knowledge of the world. Open mindsets also allow for creativity and play, which help people discover and build new skills. The broadening caused by positive emotions also leads to connection with others and better relationships. Good feelings let early humans know that it was safe to broaden and build their resources, which allowed them to flourish and better prepare themselves to survive future threats.

Compared to negative emotions which have an obvious utility, positive emotions were once considered trivial. They are not. Research shows that positive emotions are helpful and functional, and are resources that can be used in the pursuit of other important outcomes (Diener, & Biswas-Diener, 2008). Fredrickson uses the word "positivity" as an encompassing word to refer to a wide range of positive emotions including love, gratitude, interest, joy, hope, amusement, pride, inspiration, awe, and serenity. All of these emotions broaden our outlook, which allows them to make a difference in our lives. A meta-analysis of over 300 studies of positivity, which collectively tested over 275,000 people, concluded that positivity produces success in life as much as it reflects success in life (Fredrickson, 2009). Regardless of how success is measured (e.g. marital satisfaction, salary, physical health, etc.), positivity makes a difference. This is in line with the broaden-and-build theory of positive emotions; Fredrickson's decades of research show that positive emotions are generative. Her many studies say that as positive emotions broaden the scope of our attention, they cause us to take in more information, see connections to other people and things, and be more creative. They allow us to see the big picture rather than the small details (which is what negative emotions cause us to see). When we experience positivity we see our oneness and connection to others, and think of things in terms of "we" rather than "me." Research shows that these changes have a large impact over time. It's not surprising that positivity also causes people to live longer.

Because the costs of missing the sign of a nearby predator can be catastrophic, an animal's "responses to threats and unpleasantness are faster, stronger, and harder to inhibit than responses to opportunities and pleasures" (Haidt, 2006, p. 29). This phenomenon is seen across species, and is a design principle called "negativity bias" which shows up in many areas of psychology. Psychologists find that the human mind reacts differently to negative stimuli than it does positive, because we are wired to find and react to threats, violations, and setbacks. As Benjamin Franklin remarked, "We are not so sensible of the greatest Health as of the least Sickness" (Haidt, 2006, p. 29).

We are biased to respond negatively, yet positive emotions have great benefits for life, health, and success. Also, the amount of negativity appropriate for our ancestors may not be appropriate today in a world where we are not faced with life-or-death situations as frequently. Fredrickson has found that many people have a ratio of positive to negative emotions that is not adaptive or conducive to optimal functioning in today's world. She has found that the positivity ratio is actually very important, and can determine whether a person is languishing or flourishing. The "tipping point" she refers to, above which people begin to flourish is a 3:1 ratio of positive to negative emotions (Fredrickson, 2009). Because the body responds more intensely to negative emotions, humans need three positive emotions to elevate them for every one negative emotion that depresses them. According to Fredrickson, most people's positivity ratio is closer to 2:1, and some are worse. Unnecessary negativity has many detrimental effects, and without the benefits of positivity people languish. For this reason, it is important for people to increase their positivity ratios in order to flourish.

Tips for Applying this Information

Strive for the 3:1 Ratio: It is important to remember that it is not healthy to try to eliminate negativity. Both positive and negative emotions have a purpose, and the 3:1 ratio allows all negative emotions to exist. That said, much negativity is counterproductive. A powerful way to pursue happiness is to pursue positivity each day.

Track Your Emotions Daily: The first step toward understanding the value of positive emotions and reaping the benefits is becoming more mindful of your emotions. Fredrickson recommends that people keep track of the positivity and negativity they experience through daily logs. If you do this, also keep track of what made you feel the emotions. This will shed light on what makes you "come alive" so that you can devote more time and energy to those things. Pay specific attention to positive emotions – they can be a marker of an area of growth, forecasting a trajectory of development toward flourishing.

Spend Time in Activities that Cultivate Positivity: Remember the point of Fredrickson's research findings: positive emotions nourish us, and efforts to cultivate positivity are investments in our future. Often we do not give ourselves permission to spend time engaging in activities that bring us positive emotion. However, it is a wise investment in ourselves and the world around us. Positivity is not just an end, it is a means as well.

Savor Subtle Sources of Positive Emotion: You cannot force or strong-arm positivity. Subtle and unforeseen things such as a smile or a small display of kindness are often the best triggers of positivity. Fredrickson encourages people to stay open, and "soak up these subtleties as they occur. If you choose to see them, you'll soon find that they surround you. Having found them, savor them. Keep in mind that scientific studies have shown that positive emotions need not be intense or protracted to be powerful" (Fredrickson, 2009, p. 221). The key is that they be sincere and heartfelt.

Search for the Silver Lining: Fredrickson believes that it is possible to find positive meaning in any situation. Habits of thought have a large impact on well-being, and by finding positive meaning in events more frequently people raise their positivity ratio and form healthy habitual cognitive patterns. The silver lining may be subtle, and will not necessarily neutralize an aversive situation, but as stated earlier eliminating negativity is not the goal. Studies also show that feeling a small amount of heartfelt positivity in the midst of grief helps people recover much faster (Fredrickson, 2009).

Let Yourself Dream: Visualizing future success in great detail creates reliable increases in positivity (Fredrickson, 2009). Dream freely about your future, mentally conjure the best possible outcomes, and let yourself feel the joy that those outcomes would elicit. Embody those feelings. Interestingly, visualization has been shown to activate the same brain areas that actually carrying out the visualized actions would activate. This is why visualization works for athletes. Use visualization as mental practice. It is a great way to cultivate positive emotion, and it may have other performance related benefits.

Create Positive Portfolios (Fredrickson, 2009): Choose a positive emotion you would like to cultivate, and put together a portfolio of resources that elicit that emotion. To begin, think about a time when you felt that emotion strongly. What caused it? How did it feel? Represent those memories and images through photos, songs, video clips, words, art, poetry, quotes, or any other objects that evoke the feeling or sensation you are highlighting. Assemble the portfolio with love and creativity, and treat it as a gift to yourself. Engaging mindfully with the purpose of cultivating and experiencing the emotion you seek can fend off a downward spiral or help you ride a wave of positivity. Keep the portfolio alive, adding to it regularly and allowing it to evolve. This will keep your experience with it fresh. By making multiple portfolios for different emotions you can rotate them, using one predominantly and then switching subjects so that none become stale.

Meditate: Meditation is a practice that cultivates optimal states of psychological well-being and consciousness, and is a powerful positive intervention. It increases awareness and insight, and trains the mind toward optimal states of empathy, joy, and compassion. Fredrickson's research, and that of other researchers, has shown meditation to produce large boosts in positive emotion (Fredrickson, 2009). Professor Jonathan Haidt wrote, "Suppose you read about a pill that you could take once a day to reduce anxiety and increase your contentment. Would you take it? Suppose further that the pill has a great variety of side effects, all of them good: increased self-esteem, empathy, and trust; it even improves your memory. Suppose, finally, that the pill is all natural and costs nothing. Now would you take it? The pill exists. It is meditation" (Haidt, 2006, p. 35). If psychological strengths are habits of thought and being, meditation can be considered a practice of forming good habits for life. There are many styles and methods of meditation, so start exploring and experimenting with different practices. There are countless podcasts, books, recordings, and classes that can help you get started or deepen an existing practice.

<u>**Flow**</u>

Mihaly Csikszentmihalyi is a celebrated academic who has performed extensive research on consciousness and its capabilities. He argues, "the simple truth – that the control of consciousness determines the quality of life – has been known for a long time; in fact, for as long as human records exist" (Csikszentmihalyi, 2008, p. 20). That is, personal and professional satisfaction can be attained by re-ordering thoughts and actions to achieve order in consciousness. He has proposed a definition of optimal experience, which he calls "flow," and provides suggestions for how to achieve this state.

Without consciousness humans would only be able to react instinctively to circumstances. Consciousness allows people to determine the amount of joy or misery they experience, relying less on outside circumstances to do so. People have the ability to control their consciousness such that each experience is felt in a way that generates the most well-being. They must first understand the scientific aspects of the mind, how consciousness works, and then how to control it.

The flow state, or optimal experience, is achieved when there is order in consciousness. It is a state of consciousness in which a person is so immersed in what he or she is doing that nothing else seems to matter. Psychic energy is focused on something specific, and skill has met opportunity. It involves a challenge, which helps make the person engaged and focused. Csikszentmihalyi describes the state, "When all a person's relevant skills are needed to cope with the challenges of a situation, that person's attention is completely absorbed by the activity" (Csikszentmihalyi, 2008, p. 53). The experience of flow is positive and produces feelings of enjoyment. It also allows for optimal performance, personal growth, and skill development. Csikszentmihalyi argues that the most enjoyable moments in life occur during flow. Regardless of the adverse circumstances people face, anyone can adjust and eventually experience flow again. All people have the ability to experience flow, regardless of health, wealth, etc.

Disorder in consciousness is called "psychic entropy." Rage, pain, fear, anxiety, and jealousy all divert psychic energy from one's intentions, making attention unwieldy and ineffective. Also, when the mind has no demands for attention, it will wander and often land on the most problematic thoughts available. People end up using things like television to occupy their consciousness so that this does not happen, though Csikszentmihalyi advises against this strategy.   "Although average Americans have plenty of free time, and ample access to leisure activities, they do not, as a result, experience flow often" (Csikszentmihalyi, 2008, p. 83).   When left to one's own devices, there is often a void of activity, interest, and purpose that makes people unhappy. Work can be a forum in which people feel most fulfilled and happy, if they are challenged, their skills are tested, and their minds are engaged such that they achieve flow.

Goals provide purpose and help people achieve flow. Csikszentmihalyi argues that having a goal to which to direct psychic energy creates meaning. Developing this life goal is like developing a life theme. Harmony can be created by having an ultimate goal in mind, and striving to achieve flow while accomplishing the goal and its sub-goals (which make life ordered and meaningful).   Few people are satisfied simply floating through life. Through positive accomplishment, setting goals, and receiving feedback, people can live an ordered and meaningful life in flow, and simultaneously live up to their highest potential for success.

Elements of the Flow Experience:

- A Clear Goal

- Challenges Match Skills

- Concentration and Focus

- Performance Feedback

- Loss of Self-Consciousness

- Transformation of Time

<u>Tips for Working with Flow</u>

Set High-Quality Goals: See the goals section of this reference manual for information on how to set high-quality goals and get direct and immediate progress feedback.

Challenge Yourself: Being challenged helps people achieve the flow state. However, it is important to make the challenge manageable. If the activity is not challenging enough, set a higher goal. If it's too challenging, break the work into sub-goals or work on mastering the necessary skills.

Get Rid of Distractions: Put yourself in a place without distractions so that you can concentrate and focus on the goal. Also, do not think about trying to be in flow. Once you are in flow you will not be thinking about it. Rather, you will be immersed in what you are doing.

Examine Your Flow Experiences: Examine the amount of flow you experience in different areas of your life, including work, sports, hobbies, relationships, daily activities, etc. Determine when you are in flow the most, and use that information to make yourself experience more flow. You can attempt to cultivate more of the experiences that are already flow producing, or create flow in previously mundane activities.

<u>**Goal-Setting**</u>

A goal is the object or aim of an action. Goals can be set through conscious choice, and can span the length of a lifetime. Goals are important for performance in many ways: they affect the direction of a person's action, the degree of effort exerted, and the persistence of action over time (Locke, 1996). Also, they often stimulate planning, promote clarity, and enhance a person's interest in a task. Research has provided a great deal of information about the types of goals that are most effective at motivating high performance. When applying this information it is always important to keep personal context in mind. An individual's values and abilities are very important factors in his or her goal-setting process.

Higher Goals Lead to Greater Achievement: If a person is committed and possesses the prerequisite knowledge and ability to achieve a goal, then the higher the goal they set the greater their achievement will be (Latham, & Locke, 2006). This is because the effort people exert is proportional to the perceived difficulty of the goal. Harder goals also motivate greater persistence because greater persistence is often required to achieve them. When applying this research finding, it is important to be sure that goals are not set so high that they are unattainable. It is important to balance difficulty and achievability, and to be sure that an individual has the prerequisite abilities necessary to achieve any goal he or she sets.

Specific Goals Lead to Greater Achievement: The more specific and explicit a goal, the more precisely performance is regulated. Vague goals may be compatible with low performance if they are not specific and defined to require high performance.

Accomplishing Specific and Difficult Goals Requires Commitment: High levels of commitment are most important when goals are specific and difficult (Locke, 1996). High commitment requires the individual to believe the goal is important and attainable. To generate commitment adjust the goal to the individual's capacity, raise the individual's capacity through training and experience, or change the individual's perception of their capacity through expressions of confidence or role-modeling.

Goal-Setting is Most Effective When There is Progress Feedback: It is important to have performance feedback that shows a person their progress in relation to their goal. Performance feedback works best when people use it to set new goals and sub-goals. It is important that a person maintains their self-efficacy after receiving negative performance feedback. People who are able to sustain their self-efficacy tend to work harder to find improved strategies, maintain or raise their goals, and retain their commitment (Locke, 1996). People who lose their self-efficacy, or their belief that they can accomplish the goal, decrease their effort and effectiveness, and often lower their goals.

<u>Motivation</u>

There are three types of motivating forces:
1) Biological drives.
2) External forces.
3) Internal forces.

Biological drives include those for food, water, sex, etc. External motivating forces, or extrinsic motivators, usually take the form of rewards and punishments. "Carrots and sticks," or external rewards and punishments are often the primary forces used to motivate people. However, there is evidence that intrinsic motivation, motivation that comes from the inherent satisfaction of completing the task, is more effective in many circumstances.

Carrots and sticks, or "if-then" rewards and punishments, work well to motivate people to do rule-based and routine tasks. However they have downsides as well. "Traditional 'if-then' rewards can give us less of what we want: They can extinguish intrinsic motivation, diminish performance, crush creativity, and crowd out good behavior. They can also give us more of what we don't want: They can encourage unethical behavior, create addictions, and foster short-term thinking" (Pink, 2009, p. 205). Crude incentives work for simple tasks because they get people's attention and make them work hard. If the path is laid out and a task only involves mechanical skill, then a person can race to complete the task for a reward. However, crude incentives cause people to miss lateral signals, making them much worse at creative tasks and tasks that require anything more than rudimentary cognitive effort. Research shows again and again that higher incentives actually lead to worse performance on complex tasks that require conceptual thinking or creativity. Extrinsic motivators, or if-then incentives improve performance on menial tasks, but not on more complex tasks. They cause a myopia that inhibits critical thinking and creativity, and they undermine intrinsic motivation (Wiechman, & Gurland, 2009).

Fortunately, people can be powerfully motivated by the

inherent satisfaction of an activity, and intrinsic motivators can lead to the highest levels of performance and satisfaction. Intrinsic motivation is powered by the interest, joy, and purpose people feel when completing certain tasks. Furthermore, intrinsic motivation can be cultivated. Research suggests that there are three elements to intrinsic, or true motivation: *autonomy*, *mastery*, and *purpose* (Pink, 2009). Humans have an innate need to direct their own lives, learn and create new things, and connect with a purpose larger than themselves.

Autonomy

People need autonomy over:

- Task: What they do.

- Time: When they do it.

- Team: Who they do it with.

- Technique: How they do it.

(Pink, 2009)

Mastery

(Becoming better at something that matters).

- Mastery requires engagement, effort, grit, and deliberate practice.

- "Mastery begins with 'flow' – optimal experiences when the challenges we face are exquisitely matched to our abilities" (Pink, 2009, p. 207).

- Mastery requires a person to see his or her abilities as infinitely improvable.

Purpose

Purpose is often defined as a cause that is greater and more enduring than oneself.

- "Humans, by their nature, seek purpose" (Pink, 2009, p. 208).

- Group selection theory provides an evolutionary explanation for humans' desire to connect with larger goals and purpose (Haidt, 2006).

<u>Cultivating Intrinsic Motivation: Tips from Drive by Dan Pink</u>
(Pink, 2009)

Your Life in a Sentence: Contemplate your purpose by imagining that you have achieved everything you hope to in life. If someone were to describe your life and accomplishments in one simple sentence, what would they say about you? Example: Franklin Roosevelt's sentence would be, "He lifted us out of a great depression and helped us win a world war" (Pink, 2009, p.154).

Practice and Stretch: Work toward mastery and improve your performance by engaging in deliberate practice. As you improve, continually set new goals that encourage you to reach a bit higher each time. Deliberate practice is necessary for improving performance, but practice will not be maximally beneficial unless you stretch yourself.

Seek Feedback: Help yourself improve by obtaining constant, critical feedback on your progress. This will help you understand what you need to do to improve.

Explore Autonomy: Think about times when you have done your best work, what aspects of autonomy contributed to your high performance? Did you have autonomy over the task, time, technique, or team you worked with? Which aspects of autonomy are most important to you and why? How much autonomy do you have in the tasks you do in your career and personal life? To which areas would you like to bring more autonomy, and how could you go about doing so?

Break Down Barriers: Are there things you have wanted to master but have not because you are convinced that it is not possible or practical to do so? What are the barriers to engaging in these tasks? And how can you remove them?

Self-Regulation

Self-regulation is a highly adaptive and distinctively human trait that enables people to override and alter their responses, allowing individuals to take actions that live up to social and other standards (Baumeister, Gailliot, DeWall, and Oaten, 2006). Self-regulation is considered by some to be a "master virtue," for it allows people to control and improve many other areas of their lives. Baumeister et al. explain, "The ability to alter one's responses so as to bring them into line with ideals, moral values, social norms, laws, and other standards is an important key to success in life" (Baumeister et al., 2006, p. 1796). Fortunately, research suggests that it is possible to increase self-regulatory capacities through deliberate practice.

Current research indicates that self-regulation consumes a limited source, akin to an energy or strength, which is used to interrupt the stream of behavior and alter it (Baumeister et al., 2006). This energy or strength can be used up, resulting in a state that Baumeister and colleagues call "ego-depletion." There is evidence that regular exercises in self-regulation can strengthen self-regulatory abilities, or create more of this energy resource, making people less vulnerable to ego-depletion. A good analogy that is used to describe this phenomenon is the "muscle analogy." Self-regulation requires a certain amount of muscle to override and change one's actions or responses, and after being exerted muscles can become fatigued. However, with practice and consistent use, muscles strengthen and become fatigued less easily.

The fact that self-regulational abilities rely on a single core capacity has important implications, one of which is that exercises to improve self-regulation in one sphere can improve self-regulation in other spheres. Research has shown this to be true, providing evidence that consistent regulatory exercise causes wide-ranging improvements in self-control. For example, studies showed that enrolling in and complying with physical exercise programs involving 2 months of regular effort improved people's capacity for self-regulation in spheres unrelated to exercise. Participants voluntarily lessened their psychoactive substance use, compulsive spending, and even improved domestic habits such as keeping their houses clean and washing dishes. In another study, creating and following a money management plan that included keeping a spending diary and other logs again improved self-regulation with regard to psychoactive substance use, healthy eating, emotional control, maintenance of household chores, etc. Practicing self-control through improved study habits and other methods showed similar results.

Scientific evidence demonstrates that self-regulatory abilities can be improved and strengthened. Baumeister wrote, "It is possible to make the self stronger and thereby increase its ability to rise above situational demands to guide behavior" (Baumeister et al., 2006). Through regular self-regulatory exercise, people can build their self-regulatory resources and abilities. However, ego-depletion is an important factor to consider when attempting to build self-regulatory resources. Studies show that when self-regulatory resources are depleted, non-optimal inner motivations exert a greater influence on behavior. For example, a dieter who has been too strict and used up their self-regulatory resources may succumb to excessive eating.

Fortunately, there are ways to recover from ego-depletion. The work of Tice, Baumeister, Shmueli, and Muraven suggests that experiencing positive emotion restores self-regulatory resources (or "muscle"), helping the self reassert its volitional powers. A number of experiments, employing a variety of manipulations all show that positive mood or emotion counteracts ego-depletion (Tice, Baumeister, Shmueli, and Muraven, 2006). For example, after performing acts of self-regulation participants whose moods were elevated through a manipulation (watching stand-up comedy or receiving surprise gifts) did just as well on self-regulatory tasks as participants who were not previously depleted. The participants who experienced positive emotion did significantly better than participants who experienced negative emotions, neutral emotions, or had a brief rest period. Explanations for these findings may lie in Barbara Fredrickson's research, which shows that positive emotions can undo many harmful psychological effects of negative emotions.

<u>Tips for Applying this Information</u>

Strengthen Your Self-Discipline Through Exercise: Take small steps to exert self-control in many areas. Make an effort to stand up straighter, wash the dishes sooner, or exercise more. Remember as you take these small steps that you are strengthening a core reserve of self-discipline, and the effects will be far-reaching. Another approach is to make a list of beneficial habits you would like to adopt. The self-discipline practice required to adopt a new habit will affect many habits. To tackle larger issues, make reasonable plans and stick to them.

Slow and Steady Wins the Race: Attempts to be too strict when self-regulating often backfire, as ego-depletion can cause people to succumb to non-optimal inner motivations. Using the muscle analogy, overworking can cause injury. It takes time to change habits, and it takes time to strengthen the self-regulatory muscle. Set achievable goals, and acknowledge the value of small changes and diligence over time.

Remember to Re-Charge Using Positive Emotions: Non-optimal actions taken during states of ego-depletion can undo the progress made through successful self-regulation. Thus it is important to restore self-regulational resources when attempting to strengthen self-regulatory abilities. The key to this is cultivating positive emotion. Make a list of activities that elicit positive emotion, and use items on that list to reward yourself and recharge after successful self-regulation (i.e. dancing, watching comedy, playing with pets, watching sports, surfing, etc.).

Remove Temptation: Do not unnecessarily waste your

willpower. Be smart about how you use your reserves, and remove sources of temptation that will drain you.

Restore Glucose Levels: Acts of self-control deplete glucose levels, and studies have shown that restoring glucose to a sufficient level typically improves self-control (Gailliot & Baumeister, 2007). If you engage in a task that requires a great deal of self-control, eat something small afterwards that will raise your glucose levels such as fruit, rice, bread, etc.

<u>**Altruism and Giving**</u>

Research suggests that practicing acts of kindness and altruism is good for the giver as well as the recipient; being generous makes people happy (Lyubomirsky, 2008). Performing reasonable altruistic behaviors, or providing support to others that is not overtaxing, has been consistently shown to increase health and well-being (Post, & Neimark, 2007). Stephen Post, a researcher and expert on the subject, summarizes the phenomena: "Altruism results in deeper and more positive social integration, distraction from personal problems and the anxiety of self-preoccupation, enhanced meaning and purpose as related to well-being, a more active lifestyle that counters cultural pressures toward isolated passivity, and the presence of positive emotions such as kindness that displace harmful negative emotional states" (Post, 2005, p.70).

At a basic physical level, engaging in helping and self-forgetful activities, and experiencing the emotions they bring, has been shown to increase immune function and decelerate aging (Post, 2005). At an emotional and spiritual level, it is argued that generosity and other-regarding emotions bring people closer to their true and healthiest nature prescribed by moral and spiritual traditions. Other-regarding emotions and behaviors are essential to connecting with others and a higher purpose, and form the foundations of health, satisfaction, and well-being.

Evolutionary psychology provides one explanation for this association between altruism and health, well-being, and true satisfaction. Group selection theory explains that altruistic tendencies within groups are genetically selected for, because pro-social tendencies within a group create a competitive advantage over other groups in which selfishness dominates (Post, 2005). Because altruistic tendencies are evolutionarily adaptive, feelings of joy, meaning, and purpose have evolved as an emotional result of generosity to encourage altruistic behaviors and connection with others (Vaillant, 2008).

Though there is overwhelming evidence that altruistic

emotions and behaviors are healthy and contribute to well-being, there is an important caveat: there are clear adverse physical and mental health consequences of being overtaxed by altruistic behaviors (Post, 2005). The links between altruism and well-being are only present when the altruism is "reasonable." Reasonable altruism is helping behavior that is not overwhelming. It seems that the benefits of giving follow the graph of a bell curve—giving is beneficial to well-being up to a certain point, beyond which increased giving is less beneficial and can even be harmful. It is important for people to understand this, for it is up to each individual to determine the amount of giving that is healthiest for them.

Tips for Applying this Information

Help Others When You're Struggling: Performing kind acts can provide a distraction from one's own troubles, and encourages awareness and appreciation of one's good fortune. Helping others has also been shown to boost self-perception, confidence, optimism, and feelings of usefulness (Lyubomirsky, 2008). Shifting focus to others through giving can be especially helpful to people when they are experiencing emotional difficulty. However, when attempting to employ this strategy be aware of your emotional state and energy levels, and do not engage in helping behaviors if they are too taxing. Only engage in helping behaviors if you have the energy and ability, and if you see positive emotional outcomes from doing so.

Designate a Day of Kindness: Spreading small kind acts over a large time period may diminish their prominence enough that they do not have a significant impact on well-being. Create a kindness day on a regular basis in which you significantly raise your kindness level above its normal level. This could be a day of volunteering or of many kind acts.

Use Your Strengths: Help others in a way that utilizes your personal resources, abilities, interests, and expertise. This will increase your enjoyment and engagement in the task, help you make a more significant impact, and contribute to the feelings of usefulness and self-esteem that giving cultivates.

Count Kindness: Develop an eye and appreciation for kindness. By noticing more kindness you'll experience more of it in your life. Counting kindness interventions involve taking daily tallies (mental or physical) of kind acts committed and witnessed, and have been shown to increase people's levels of positivity (Fredrickson, 2009).   Also, witnessing and hearing about kindness has been shown to emotionally elevate people and increase their desire to do good deeds (Lyubomirsky, 2008). Shine the light of your attention on the kindness that is already around you, and experience the benefits that kindness has on well-being.

Keep it Fresh: Variety allows helping behaviors to continue to feel extraordinary and meaningful over time. New and special acts that help you rise above your daily kindness routine can be very helpful, such as donating your time, surprising someone with a nice gesture, offering a sincere smile, or developing compassion for others by trying to see things from their point of view.

Let Go of Ego and the Desire for Recognition: Resolve not to judge others for not doing good deeds, and also resolve not to do these good deeds for approval or admiration (Lyubomirsky, 2008). This will deepen the sense of meaning, value, and self-worth you gain. Perhaps do a deed about which you tell no one and expect nothing in return.

Remember that Giving is not Always Beneficial: As discussed earlier, kindness is not beneficial when it is overtaxing to the giver. Helping behavior that is burdensome or interferes with daily goals and functioning actually has a negative impact on well-being. Also, kind acts need to be done freely and autonomously to be maximally beneficial. Forcing others to engage in altruistic behaviors may not be helpful to them, and may even cause bitterness. Lastly, *helping is not always beneficial to the person receiving the "help."* It can make people feel needy, disadvantaged, or beholden (Lyubomirsky, 2008). Keep this in mind and stay attuned to the situation as you try to help others. Be mindful of how your attitude affects those you are helping, and be sure that they want your help. Do not help those who do not want your help.

Gratitude

Gratitude is a commonly experienced emotion, and it can also represent an attitude or a tendency to see life as a gift. Expressing and experiencing gratitude generates many positive outcomes, including peace of mind, satisfying personal relationships, and happiness in general. Gratitude is valued ubiquitously across many cultures, and is almost universally considered a virtue. It is easy to understand why noticing and appreciating the positive elements of one's life improves well-being, and there is a great deal of scientific evidence suggesting that gratitude has a causal influence on subjective well-being (Giacomo, Emmons, and McCullough, 2004). Research has shown gratitude to be a powerful force for creating positive changes in individuals, families, and organizations. In fact, according to Sonja Lyubomirsky, a researcher professor of Psychology, "The expression of gratitude is a kind of metastrategy for achieving happiness" (Lyubomirsky, 2008, p.89). However, gratitude does not always come naturally, and is a virtue that can and must be cultivated. Thus, the field of positive psychology includes many interventions that help people feel thankful for the gifts they experience in their lives.

Ways that Gratitude Boosts Happiness (Lyubomirsky, 2008):

- Promotes savoring of the gifts one experiences in life.

- Bolsters self-worth and self-esteem.

- Encourages moral behavior.

- Helps people cope with stress, trauma, and adversity.

- Helps build social bonds.

- Inhibits negative comparisons with others.

- Pushes out and replaces negative emotions.

- Thwarts hedonic adaptation, or our ability to rapidly adjust to new positive circumstances.

Research has shown that interventions can effectively increase gratitude and the positive benefits of gratitude. This is true for a wide range of populations. Gratitude can be measured in intensity (for a positive event), frequency (number of times felt throughout a day), span (scope of things for which someone is grateful at any given time), and density (gratitude toward more people or things for an event) (Giacomo et al., 2004).

Tips for Applying this Information

Ritualize Gratitude: Make gratitude an active component of your daily routine. Keeping a gratitude journal, sharing positive events with a gratitude partner, expressing gratitude before meals, or taking a moment during endings to acknowledge and appreciate the goodness that transpired can become part of a healthy gratitude practice (Fredrickson, 2009).

Gratitude Journal: Write down what you are grateful for each day, and describe in detail why each good thing happened. This draws the attention to the precursors of good events and helps people become aware of more things to be grateful for, deepening the experience.

Gratitude Essay or Letter: Write an essay about, or a letter to someone to whom you feel grateful. Explain why you feel grateful in detail. If you write a letter it is not necessary to deliver it, but delivering it can produce even more positive emotion for the writer and the receiver.

Gratitude Partner: Plan to practice gratitude regularly with a partner by sharing good news and discussing things you feel grateful for. Respond actively and constructively when your partner shares, feeling the joy and gratitude with them when they share their blessings.

Meditate on the Feeling of Gratitude: Sit in a quiet place to meditate. Incorporate gratitude practice into your meditation by continually calling to mind things you feel grateful for. When the feeling of gratitude comes, focus all of your attention on it. Experience the feeling of gratitude throughout your entire body. Continue in this way, calling to mind things you feel grateful for and meditating on the experience of the grateful feelings that come.

Express Gratitude Directly: Make a habit of thanking people authentically for the things they do for you and the impact they have on your life. Be aware of the kindness of others and acknowledge it. This practice can bring positive emotion to both of you.

Gratitude Portfolio: Make a portfolio of things that make you feel grateful. It can include pictures, poems, artifacts, memories, and anything else that elicits the emotion of gratitude. Spend time on it and make it beautiful. Both working on the portfolio and reviewing what you have made will cultivate grateful feelings. Keep the portfolio living and add to it from time to time to keep the experience you have with it fresh.

Ritualize Endings: Researcher Barbara Fredrickson takes time to acknowledge endings, large and small, and cultivate gratitude for the goodness that transpired before moving forward. If she's with people, she thanks them aloud or shares her grateful feelings with them. Little endings happen all the time, and each one can be a cue to give thanks in a new and unique way (Fredrickson, 2009).

Vary Your Techniques and Keep Your Gratitude Practice Fresh: Do not over-practice or attempt to use the same gratitude strategy in the same way over and over. A practice will not elicit gratitude if it becomes stale.

<u>**Savoring**</u>

The way people experience positive events determines how much positive emotion the event will generate, and how much it will promote their well-being. "The active management of positive emotion requires, not only the capacity to feel pleasure, but also, the capacity to regulate it, to find it, to manipulate it, and to sustain it" (Bryant, 2003, p. 176). Savoring is a process that allows people to improve the frequency, intensity, and duration of the positive emotions they experience. It "requires a mindful awareness of enjoyment, a deliberate conscious attention to the experience of pleasure" (Bryant, 2003, p. 195). Savoring consists of intentionally engaging in thoughts and behaviors that heighten the positive emotions that a pleasurable experience elicits (Reivich, 2010). This form of control of positive emotions positively correlates with a number of beneficial qualities including optimism, high self-esteem, high life satisfaction, internal locus of control, etc. It negatively correlates with qualities such as neuroticism, depression, and guilt. Savoring is a powerful strategy for cultivating engagement, meaning, positive emotion, gratitude, and mindfulness (Reivich, 2010).

It is possible to savor by reflecting on an event cognitively or by losing oneself in the moment experientially. Also, rather than merely reacting to positive events when they happen to occur, people can "learn to savour proactively – to consciously anticipate positive experiences, to mindfully accentuate and sustain pleasurable moments, and to deliberately remember these experiences in ways that rekindle enjoyment after they end" (Bryant, 2003, p. 195).

There are three temporal orientations through which people can savor (Bryant, 2003):

Anticipation: Generating positive feelings before an event occurs.

Present enjoyment: Generating positive feelings in the present by intensifying or prolonging them through thoughts and behaviors.

Reminiscence: Generating positive feelings by looking back on an event in a way that re-kindles positive emotion.

There are four types of savoring (Seligman, 2002):

Basking: Reveling in or making the most of praise or congratulations.

Thanksgiving: Experiencing or expressing gratitude.

Marveling: Being filled with wonder, astonishment, or awe.

Luxuriating: Delighting in the experience of the senses.

<u>Tips for Applying this Information</u>

Examine Beliefs About Enjoyment and Savoring: Examine your beliefs about your ability to control the amount of pleasure you receive from events. If you believe you can maximize the amount of positive emotion you feel through processes like savoring, you are in a great place – move forward. If you find that you hold beliefs about an inability to experience positive emotion, look to the Resilience Skills section of this reference manual and work on challenging those beliefs. Also, delve further into the research evidence regarding the benefits of savoring. Remove hindrances to your experience of positive emotion by examining any beliefs that may be getting in the way.

Explore the Ways You Currently Savor: Think about when you savor, and how. Compare what you do to the four types and three temporal forms. In which areas would you like to savor more? It is possible to learn to anticipate, reminisce, and savor the moment more effectively, and it is also possible to choose to bask, marvel, be thankful, and luxuriate more. Become conscious of how you currently savor, and the ways you would like to savor more.

Share with Others: Capitalize! Share your joy and appreciation with others, and express your gratitude. (See the Active-Constructive Responding section)

Actively Build Memories: Take mental or physical notes and photographs and reflect on them later. Doing so makes it easier to reflect upon and remember the joy of an experience.

Express Pleasant Feelings Behaviorally: Laugh, jump for joy, etc.

Sharpen Sensory Perceptions: Intensify pleasure by focusing on certain sensory stimuli and screening out others (Seligman, 2002).

Immerse Yourself in the Moment: Let the meaning you attach to your thoughts go, and become completely absorbed in the experience of the present moment.

<u>Hope</u>

Individuals experience hope when they expect or believe that a desired goal can be achieved (Feudtner, 2010). Hope is a positive outcome itself, but it also has benefits via the positive emotions it produces. In addition, it improves the timing and quality of decisions and actions, and helps sustain motivation (Feudtner, 2005). "Higher hope consistently is related to better outcomes in academics, athletics, physical health, psychological adjustment, and psychotherapy" (Snyder, 2002, p. 249). Highly hopeful thinking is also accompanied by trait-like emotional states or moods, which set the affective tone of the goal pursuit (Snyder, 2002). High hope corresponds to enduring positive emotions and traits such as zest, friendliness, happiness, and confidence. Low hope corresponds to lethargy and negative or passive emotions related to goal pursuit. People who are high in hope cope better and are less likely to view impediments to goals as stressful. They also generate more goals, and are more likely to select goals that stretch them.

Hope has three essential components:
1) Goals.
2) Pathway Thoughts ("Way Power").
3) Agency Thoughts ("Will Power") (Snyder, 2002).

Goals provide the targets for cognitive processes. People approach goal pursuits by generating routes to achieving the goals, which are the pathways. People who are high in hope are good at generating pathways, particularly alternative pathways when their goal pursuits are impeded. Pathway thinking becomes increasingly precise and refined as people near their goal. Agency thought is a person's perceived capacity to achieve their goal through the pathways. Agency beliefs and the self-talk they produce can create the motivation necessary for people to pursue the pathways to their goals and succeed. Hope can be explicitly and skillfully managed by manipulating these three elements of hope. This can facilitate transformations in the way individuals think and feel about their situation, which has a direct impact on the decisions they make and their experience of life (Feudtner, 2005).

Tips for Accentuating Hope

Re-Goaling: At times it is important to explicitly revisit a person's hopes, and ask whether or not it is time to emphasize different goals. When hope for a major dream is destroyed, it is possible to regenerate hope by setting different goals (Feudtner, 2010). "Bad news" can threaten certain hopes, but it can be used to reorient individuals toward other hopes. At times when hope seems lost, look at the goals and ask how hopes are faring. If they are not doing well, and it seems that it is time to emphasize different goals, ask what the individual does have to be hopeful for given the circumstances. Create new goals based on the response.

Augment Agency Thoughts: People who are high in hope engage in positive self-talk beginning at the outset of a goal task, and they maintain their positive attitude (Snyder, 2002). Be aware of the thoughts you think about your ability to accomplish your goals. Thoughts like, "I'm ready for this challenge," or "This will be interesting, maybe even fun," elicit positive emotions that reinforce the agency aspect of the hope trilogy, enhancing motivation and persistence.

Cultivate Positive Emotion: Positive and negative emotions feed into a person's agency thoughts, even if the emotions are elicited by events outside the goal directed process (Snyder, 2002). Negative feelings cue self-critical rumination, and can cause people's cognitions to lose focus from the task. It is best to stay in a hopeful and positive space while attempting goal pursuits. If this is not possible, take a break from the goal process and attempt to generate positive emotion in another way. When you return to the goal pursuit, the positive emotion will translate and provide more hope and better outcomes in the goal pursuit (Snyder, 2002).

Surround Yourself with Hopeful People: Hope is learned, and mostly in the context of other people. The social network of relationships is very important because it impacts the goals that are formed and how hope is cast. Remember that hope does not occur in a vacuum, so surround yourself with hopeful, goal-directed people who support your hope.

Expand Your Pathway Thought Repertoire: Remind yourself of the fact that your goals can be achieved through many feasible avenues. Get creative, generate action scenarios, and sketch out the possibilities.

<u>**Active Constructive Responding**</u>

Capitalization is the act of sharing news of a positive event with another. Professor Shelly Gable has done a great deal of research on communication and relationships, and has found that partners' responses to capitalization attempts are very important to relationship health and satisfaction. Partners' responses to capitalization attempts correlate with relationship commitment, satisfaction, and love (Gable, Gonzaga, and Strachman, 2006). They are also more closely related to relationship well-being and break-ups than are partners' responses to negative event discussions. This means that the way a person responds when their partner shares good news matters a great deal, and is likely to matter more to a relationship's health than when their partner shares bad news. Gable has categorized types of responses to capitalization attempts, and her findings provide valuable information about the style of communication that is healthiest for relationships. She categorizes the best types of responses as both 'active' and 'constructive.' Active constructive responding (ACR) is a powerful positive intervention and is beneficial for all relationships, not just romantic relationships.

<u>The Four Types of Responses</u>

Active Constructive: Authentic, enthusiastic support

- Feeling the joy along with the person who is sharing.

- Often involves asking for details and helping the capitalizer savor the news.

- Example: "That's wonderful news. I'm so happy for you! Tell me more about it."

Passive Constructive: Quiet, understated support

- Does not show much excitement or interest in the capitalizer's good news.

- Example: "That's nice dear."

Active Destructive: Demeaning or quashing the news

- Making critical, negative, or pessimistic remarks about the information that was shared.

- Example: "That's never going to work out. It'll probably add a lot of stress in your life."

Passive Destructive: Ignoring the event

- Does not acknowledge the capitalizer's news or feelings about the news at all.

- Example: "So anyway…Guess what happened to me at work today."

Research shows that people who rate their partners as active and constructive responders feel more intimacy and trust, are more satisfied with the relationship, report fewer conflicts, and engage in more fun and relaxing activities together (Gable et al., 2006). This is because active constructive responding makes people feel validated, understood, and cared for. Active and constructive responses confirm the importance of the positive event and help elaborate on it. Passive or destructive responses may imply that the responder does not think the news is important, or that they do not understand or care about what is important to the capitalizer.

<u>Tips for Applying this Information</u>

Explore Your Response Style: How do you normally respond when people in your life share good news? Do you have a habitual style? Do you have different response styles with different people? How does your response style affect your relationships?

Use More ACR: Once you are aware of your response style, attempt to use more ACR. Make a point of celebrating good news with the people in your life, and see the difference it makes in your relationships.

Capitalize More: Communicating personal positive events with others is associated with increased positive affect and well-being (Gable, Asher, Reis, & Impett, 2004). Take note of the response styles of the people around you, and make attempts to capitalize more with those who respond actively and constructively to you. Encourage them to capitalize more with you as well, and return the favor. Capitalizing more increases the opportunities for people to share joy with one another, and strengthens relationships. If you find it hard to capitalize, explore the blockages you have to sharing your good news with others.

Combine Capitalizing With Gratitude Exercises: If you do gratitude exercises that involve writing down things you are grateful for, make a point of sharing some of them. Choose one item from your gratitude journal every day to share with a significant other and encourage them to do the same.

<u>**Excess Choice**</u>

Dr. Barry Schwartz' research offers insight into a peculiar problem that individuals living in modern, affluent societies face. Though people are receiving objectively better outcomes in many areas of life, they are less satisfied with those outcomes. Schwartz' compelling research links this problem to what he considers an overabundance of choice available to people in these societies. This section summarizes his research findings explaining the implications they have for well-being, and also provides tips for applying this information.

According to Schwartz, western industrial societies have deeply embedded assumptions and beliefs relating to choice that are not necessarily true. The first assumption is that the way to maximize welfare is to increase individual freedom. The second is that the way to maximize freedom is to increase choice. The logic is that given freedom and opportunity, people will make choices that maximize their well-being. Schwartz' research indicates that this may not be the case. According to him, increased choice is conducive to well-being up to a certain point, after which it becomes detrimental.

Schwartz points out that the number of available choices has exploded in many areas of life, from the number of available salad dressings and stereos, to career options, etc. If the societal assumptions were true, people would be more satisfied now that they have more options. However, according to Schwartz, "We get what we want, only to discover that what we want doesn't satisfy us to the degree that we expect" (Schwartz, 2004, p. 221). The problems with too much choice are such: too much choice causes paralysis instead of liberation, making it difficult for people to chose at all; and too much choice also causes people to be less satisfied with whatever they chose.

These claims are based in strong empirical evidence. For example, in investments in voluntary retirement plans, for every ten additional mutual funds offered by the employer the rate of employee participation decreased (Schwartz, 2004). Schwartz contends that when offered 50 mutual funds plans, people find the decision hard to make, and put it off, sometimes indefinitely. The people who do not chose at all then lose the money that would have been matched by their employer, in this case up to $5,000 per year.

Why Excess Choice Causes Dissatisfaction

Regret and Anticipated Regret: When given many choices, if something is not perfect it is easy to imagine a better alternative, and regret anything that is not perfect about the option chosen.

Opportunity Costs: After making a choice when there were many alternatives to consider, it's easy to imagine the benefits of the alternative options that were rejected. There are always benefits of alternative options that are lost when choosing an option. Even if what is chosen is perceived as preferable, the mental value of the lost benefits detracts from satisfaction with what is chosen. The more options, the greater the opportunity costs.

Escalation of Expectations: An abundance of choice makes it possible to have objectively better outcomes, but people feel worse because options raise expectations about how good the objective outcome should be. An individual's end result is then disappointing compared to their expectations. The more options the greater the increase in expectations.

Self-Blame: When a person is given many options, if the outcome is disappointing they will feel that they are at fault. Rather than blaming the lack of options, people blame themselves. Schwartz argues that this has contributed to the explosion of depression western societies have experienced.

Barry Schwartz' Tips and Suggestions for Optimizing Satisfaction in the Face of Choice
(Schwartz, 2004)

Appreciate the Costs of Decision Making: Review recent decisions you have made, large and small.   Itemize the steps, time, research, and anxiety that went into making the decisions. Focus your attention on how it felt to do the work of choosing. Finally, ask yourself how much the final decision benefited from the work. You may find that this exercise gives you incentive to limit the energy you spend making certain decisions or give up some decisions altogether.

Embrace "Satisficing":   "Maximizers" strive to make the absolute best decision. They are always looking for the next best thing, and spend a great deal of time and energy making choices. Maximizers also tend to have more depression, regret, and anxiety. "Satisficers" can accept something as "good enough." Schwartz argues that this simplifies decision-making and increases satisfaction. While someone who maximizes might obtain an objectively better outcome, they will be subjectively worse off, and less satisfied with their choice. By embracing and appreciating satisficing, and attempting to intentionally cultivate it, people have less regret and more peace of mind. To satisfice more, think about occasions when you have comfortably settled for "good enough." Think about how you made choices in those areas, and attempt to apply these strategies more broadly. Some Maximizers have strong negative reactions to this advice, declaring that they aren't willing to settle. Don't settle on the things that are important to you, but be aware of the costs of your decision-making process. With this better understanding of how satisfaction is determined, people can find the balance between satisficing and maximizing that works best for them.

Choose When to Choose: Decide which choices really need thought and effort. When it comes to the less important things, you will actually be more satisfied and happy if you spend less time deciding and let some opportunities pass you by. "Shorten or eliminate deliberations about decisions that are unimportant to you; use some of the time you've freed up to ask yourself what you really want in the areas of your life where decisions matter"

(Schwartz, 2004, p. 224).

Adopt Personal Rules and Limitations: Establish some rules of thumb for how many options you will allow yourself to consider, or how much time and energy you will spend choosing.

Make Decisions Non-Reversible: Knowing that a decision is permanent makes people work to improve the relationship they have with it, rather than constantly second-guessing their decision.

Practice Gratitude: Focus on the good elements of decisions you have made rather than focusing on the things you are disappointed with. This will help lessen regret.

Anticipate Adaptation: Humans adapt to almost everything they experience regularly. Things that initially give a person pleasure are likely to lose their luster over time. By developing realistic expectations about how experiences change with time we can prevent the dissatisfaction that often accompanies adaptation. Prepare yourself for adaptation when you buy things, knowing that they will not give you as much pleasure in a few months. When you experience adaptation, practice gratitude and remind yourself of how good things actually are, rather than comparing them to how great they felt before.

Limit Social Comparison: Social comparison often reduces people's satisfaction. There will always be someone better off than you, who has better clothing and drives a nicer car. But so what? Focus on the things that add meaning to your life and make you happy, and remember that what you have is good enough.

<u>Coaching</u>

Paralleling the growth of the field of positive psychology, the profession of coaching has been rapidly expanding over the last decade. Coaching applications are applied in many domains such as personal, health, workplace and executive settings. The International Coach Federation (ICF) defines coaching as "an ongoing professional relationship that helps people produce extraordinary results in their lives, careers, businesses, or organizations. Through the process of coaching, clients deepen their learning, improve their performance, and enhance their quality of life" (Whitworth, Kimsey-House, Kimsey-House & Sandahl, 2007, p.290). The principles of coaching, or the methodologies for helping individuals reach their goals and fulfill their potential, have been in existence for many years. Only recently has the coaching format become a popular methodology for facilitating change. As of 2011, the annual revenue expended on corporate coaching was estimated as $1.5 billion, with 30,000 professional coaches practicing globally (Sheldon, Kashdan, & Steger, 2011).

Like the field itself, the majority of the research on coaching is less than a decade old. However, there is significant research supporting its efficacy. Sheldon et. al. wrote, "The 11 randomized controlled studies of coaching that have been conducted to date indicate that coaching can indeed improve performance in various ways" (Sheldon et al., 2011, p.297). Coaching has been empirically shown to facilitate goal attainment, improve well-being and reduce stress. The 11 studies have spanned workplace, health, and personal domains, and all have had good outcomes. That said, more randomized, controlled studies are necessary to build a solid scientific understanding of the efficacy of coaching.

Coaching facilitates the process of human change through the relationship formed between the coach and coachee, helping the coachee remain focused on the goals that will enhance his or her well-being. The relationship is co-created and unique to each pair or group (yes, coaching can be a group activity), and serves the purpose of helping the client attain valued personal, professional, and health outcomes. The results are attained through the coach's help identifying desired outcomes, establishing and remaining focused on important goals over time, building motivation and action plans, and creating and implementing solutions to challenges that arise throughout the goal attainment process. In a way that is different from a typical therapeutic approach, coaching assumes that the client is naturally creative, resourceful, and whole. Another important feature of coaching is that the client sets the agenda, and the coach responds to that agenda. The coach uses skills of deep listening and asking powerful questions to forward and deepen the conversation, acting as a catalyst in the change process.

The profession of coaching is still maturing. Currently there are no barriers to entry in the field (i.e. anyone can call themselves a coach, regardless of their training, skills, and experience). The ICF, a non-profit organization, does offer credentials and accreditations and has worked to create formal ethical and practice standards. However, the practice of coaching is still largely unregulated and there is a wide range in quality, competencies, and practices within coaching professionals. This is changing with time, as coaching is becoming more accepted in academia and psychological societies. Some argue that positive psychology can provide the theoretical and scientific backbone the field is searching for. With time, it is reasonable to assume that the quality standards of coaching will continue to rise. Despite the current range in skill among coaching professionals, there are many phenomenal coaches and coach training programs that are living examples of the excellence the field is capable of attaining.

<u>**Appreciative Inquiry**</u>

Appreciative Inquiry (AI) is a methodology for promoting positive organizational change by tapping into and building upon an organization's best practices. It accomplishes this by creating a structured, meaningful dialogue designed to inspire hope and action among the organization's stakeholders. The methodology was developed over a number of years by Dr. David Cooperrider, who began developing the methodology as a student of Organizational Behavior at Case Western University in the 1980's. A paper later written by Cooperrider and Dr. Diana Whitney describes the methodology, "Appreciative Inquiry is the cooperative search for the best in people, their organizations, and the world around them. It involves systematic discovery of what gives a system "life" when it is most effective and capable in economic, ecological, and human terms. AI involves the art and practice of asking questions that strengthen a system's capacity to heighten positive potential" (Cooperrider & Whitney, 2007, p. 245-263).

AI utilizes a model of future-oriented, strength-based change unlike many organizational change processes that focus on fixing problems. Deficit based change processes can limit new images of possibility from forming and can increase hierarchical and problem-oriented language (which do not motivate or inspire). In an interesting study, Losada & Fredrickson found that high performing teams had approximately a 6:1 ratio of strength or opportunity focused dialogue to negative or deficiency focused dialogue, while low performing teams had approximately a 1:3 ratio of strength to deficiency focused dialogue (Fredrickson & Losada, 2005).

The AI process is centered around a powerfully framed affirmative topic, which is the topic (or topics) chosen in advance to be explored through the change process. Affirmative topics do not use deficit based language, but rather describe what you want to get more of through the inquiry. For example, "Low Morale" is not a powerfully framed affirmative topic. The flip side of that, "High Commitment and a Sense of Shared Ownership" could be an affirmative topic.

Another attribute of AI is that it focuses on engagement of the "whole," meaning that the process is neither top down nor bottom up; all of the organization's stakeholders are equally involved in strategic planning. The methodology uses the "art of the question" to tap into the collective intelligence of the "whole," and direct its attention. Through carefully crafted questions it creates an exploration into the positive core, or strengths of an organization. From there, questions direct the attention of the group to possibilities for the future, and guide them to design an ideal future that they'll eventually bring to life.

The process is structured around four phases of inquiry (the 4-D process):

1. Discovery: "What gives life to the organization?"

    - The Discovery phase involves an inquiry into the organization's positive core or strengths.

    - The strengths or positive core are the things that the organization will keep and expand as it changes.

2. Dream: "What might be?"

    - The Dream phase involves an unrestrained envisioning of ideal possibilities for the future (results and impact).

    - The dreams are grounded in the strengths that were discovered in phase 1.

3. Design: "What should be the ideal?"

    - The design phase involves honing in on the best possible results and impact, and co-constructing that vision.

4. Destiny: "How to empower, learn, and improvise?"

- The final phase is also sometimes referred to as "Delivery," and is the implementation stage.

Appreciative Inquiry is usually administered in the form of a summit, which can involve hundreds or even thousands of people. It requires careful planning by a team that includes representatives from as many stakeholder groups as possible. Some of the most important preparations include conducting a mini-inquiry to help choose an affirmative topic, mapping out the stakeholders, and designing the questions for each phase of the summit.

<u>Tips for Employing Appreciative Inquiry Techniques</u>

Educate and Plan: If you decide you'd like to use an AI summit to facilitate change in your organization, do not go into it unprepared. Like many powerful methodologies it takes skill and understanding to facilitate a summit, and failure to take an organization through the process correctly can be de-motivating and discouraging to participants if results are not achieved. Though the language utilized by the methodology seems light and carefree, it is a serious methodology and should be treated as such. Educate yourself and plan extensively before facilitating a summit. Ideally it is best to attend or assist the facilitation of other summits so that the first one you design is not the first one you experience. Case Western University has an excellent online portal with free resources, tools, and summit materials called the Appreciative Inquiry Commons.

Ask High-Point Questions: Appreciative Inquiry derives affirmative topics and investigates an organization's positive core through the use of high-point questions. High-point questions inquire into a high-point in a person's career or experience with the organization, and draw out a story. After getting the story, they inquire into the strengths and resources that made the high-point possible. Using high-point questions is an engaging way to explore strengths, and can be used to discover strengths in non-organizational contexts as well.

Ask Powerful Questions: People and organizations grow in the direction of their attention, and questions are an excellent tool for directing attention toward possibilities for a better future. Utilize the power of inquiry to increase clarity, action, and discovery by asking powerful questions such as, "What is your desired outcome?," "How does this relate to your life purpose?," or "What will you do to achieve this, and when will you do it?" There are a limitless number of powerful questions to be asked, so start practicing and coming up with new ones of your own.

Use the 4-D Process to Facilitate Transformation in Creative Ways: The 4-D process can be adapted and used outside of the AI summit model in coaching and other organizational endeavors. The 4-D process—discovering strengths through inquiry, brainstorming possibilities, designing best possible future outcomes, and then beginning to implement—is a powerful and elegant roadmap for transformation. For example, a coach can take an individual client through an inquiry that hits each of the four phases. Become familiar with the 4-D process, and you'll be surprised at the number of creative ways it can be used outside of a planned summit.

<u>**Resilience**</u>

Resilience refers to the ability to cope with adversity, or "persevere and adapt when things go awry" (Reivich, and Shatté, 2002, p.1). The study of resilience began as researchers started to search for and identify characteristics of individuals, mostly young people, who were able to thrive despite facing adversity and numerous risk-factors. This led to a list of resilient qualities, strengths, and protective factors that can be accessed to grow through adversity (Richardson, 2002). Resilient characteristics including happiness, subjective well-being, optimism, faith, self-determination, wisdom, creativity, self-control, and gratitude were identified by researchers. The next step in the study of resilience involved an inquiry into the process of attaining the identified resilient qualities. Finally, some resilience researchers began to explore the concept of innate resilience, described as a "motivational force within everyone that drives them to pursue wisdom, self-actualization, and altruism and to be in harmony with a spiritual source of strength" (Richardson, 2002, p. 309).

According to a Harvard Business Review's analysis of the research on resilience, resilient people possess three characteristics: "a staunch acceptance of reality; a deep belief…that life is meaningful; and an uncanny ability to improvise" (Coutu, 2002, p.48). All of these characteristics can be linked to individuals' thoughts and beliefs, which is consistent with other resilience researchers' assertion that thinking is central to resilience. Thoughts and perceptions influence the way people cope with stress and handle adversity, and certain beliefs can lead to longer, happier, and healthier lives (Reivich, and Shatté, 2002). Resilience skills can help individuals scrutinize the beliefs behind their explanations of events, and change them if necessary. Resilient thinking styles are characterized by *accurate* and *flexible* thinking, and are cultivated through increased awareness and practice. Resilience work helps people cast off negative self-image, reduce harsh self-criticism, increase optimism, navigate through challenges, and have the courage to reach out and take chances. Research has shown resilient people to be physically healthier, more successful in school and work, more satisfied with their relationships, and less prone to depression than those who do not possess resilience skills.

Elements of Resilience (Reivich, and Shatté, 2002):

- **Emotional Regulation**: The ability to control one's emotions, particularly in the face of adversity, in order to stay focused and centered.

- **Impulse Control**: The ability to control behavior under pressure.

- **Causal Analysis**: The ability to completely and accurately identify the causes of problems in order to prevent the same thing from happening again in the future.

- **Self-Efficacy**: A sense of competence and mastery in the world.

- **Realistic Optimism**: The belief that things can go well, that there is hope for the future, and that it is possible to control the course of one's own life. (These beliefs must be grounded in reality).

- **Empathy**: The ability to read and be attuned to other people's psychological and emotional states.

- **Reaching Out**: The ability to seek new opportunities, challenges, and relationships for greater satisfaction and success in life.

The first step in becoming more resilient is to become aware of the relationship between your thoughts and emotions. This will help you gain insight into your thoughts (beliefs) when things go wrong, and give you the ability to make changes in your beliefs when they cause debilitating emotional and behavioral reactions.

<u>Resilience: The ABC Process</u>

Contrary to common perception, the events in an individual's life do not cause his or her feelings and behavioral reactions. A person's thoughts and beliefs about the life events drive his or her feelings and behaviors. The first step in becoming resilient begins with self-awareness. Individuals are instructed to become aware of their mental interpretations of negative events, or their "inner monologue" when things go wrong or they experience negative emotions. Once they are aware of the thoughts that cause their emotions and reactions, they can take measures to cultivate thoughts that lead to healthy outcomes. The "ABC" process was developed by two of the world's leading cognitive therapists Dr. Steven Hollon and Dr. Arthur Freeman, along with Dr. Martin Seligman (Seligman, 1991). It is a tool that helps people become aware of their thoughts and the outcomes the thoughts have on their lives.

Any time you face an adversity, separate out the A, B, C (Seligman, 1991):

> **A= Adversity**: The activating event (the objective who, what, when, and where).
> **B= Beliefs**: Thoughts about the event (your mental dialogue).
> **C= Consequences**: Feelings and behavior (how you felt and what you did).

<u>Note that certain types of beliefs lead to specific emotional reactions:</u>

The belief that your rights have been violated → Anger

The belief that you've experienced a loss/loss of self-worth → Sadness

The belief that you've violated the rights of another → Guilt

The belief that you compare negatively to others → Embarrassment

The belief that there is a future threat → Anxiety

(Reivich, and Shatté, 2002)

Use this information to help you understand the mix of emotions you feel when faced with an adversity, and identify the types of beliefs that get you "stuck" or make you react a certain way. Once you have identified the beliefs, then you can examine them for accuracy. Begin to think about alternative ways to view the situation, and challenge inaccurate beliefs with new thoughts or interpretations that elicit more productive emotions.

Resilience: Explanatory Style

A person's explanatory style is the habitual way they explain the causes of the good and bad things that happen to them (Peterson, 1991).

Explanatory styles can be coded along three dimensions:

Personal (me - not me)

- Internal vs. external

- Example: a person automatically thinks the cause of the problem is them, OR they automatically think the cause of the problem is someone else.

Permanent (always - not always)

- Permanent vs. temporary

- Example: a person automatically thinks the problem is lasting and unchangeable, OR they see it as changeable.

Pervasive (everything - not everything)

- Specific vs. universal

- Example: a person thinks that the problem will undermine all aspects of his or her life (everything), OR that this is an isolated event.

    (Seligman, 1991)

People who have an "always-everything" explanatory style have difficulty finding solutions to their problems. People who focus on the "not always- not everything causes" are much more likely to be able to generate new solutions to their problems. However, the most resilient people do not get caught in one explanatory style, which allows them to identify all significant causes. Their thinking is flexible and therefore more accurate.

Resilience: Avoiding Cognitive Distortions

There are common thinking errors, or patterns of thought that cause beliefs and interpretations to become inaccurate. Examine your beliefs about a situation using the ABC process, and check for these errors. Over time, you may find that you tend to succumb to certain errors more than others. Notice your patterns and keep them in mind. Knowing which patterns you tend to fall into will help you stay aware and collected during the moments when adversity strikes. Cognitive distortions were initially proposed by Aaron Beck, the father of cognitive therapy. Today there are many names for the distortions, and a number of lists have been created. The following is a list of "Thinking Traps" from Reivich & Shatté's book <u>The Resilience Factor</u> (Reivich, and Shatté, 2002). Their list is a descendant of Beck's original work.

- Jumping to conclusions: Drawing conclusions (usually negative) from little evidence.

- Tunnel vision: Only seeing the negative (or positive) aspects of a situation.

- Magnifying and minimizing: Distorting aspects of a situation by maximizing or minimizing (e.g. "Making a mountain out of a molehill," or minimizing the positive).

- Personalizing: Incorrectly seeing oneself as the cause of an event.

- Externalizing: Incorrectly attributing the cause of events to external agents.

- Overgeneralizing: Making wide generalizations from isolated events.

- Mind reading: Presuming to know the intentions and thoughts of others.

- Emotional reasoning: Assuming that one's negative emotions are accurate gauges of a situation, or making decisions based on feeling rather than evidence and reason.

<u>Resilience: Disputation and Distraction</u>

Disputation and distraction are the "D" category that is added on to the "ABC" process (Seligman, 1991). The ABC process allows people to become aware of the thoughts or beliefs that are not serving them, and disputation and distraction are processes for dealing with those thoughts most effectively. When a person is experiencing destructive or pessimistic thoughts, the first option they have is to distract themselves and attempt to place their thoughts and attention on more productive things. The second option is to dispute the negative thoughts, which is more effective because it makes the thoughts less likely to occur in the future (Seligman, 1991).

Distraction is an important tool for breaking the cycle of rumination. One method is to physically interrupt the chain of thoughts. This can involve ringing a bell, writing the word STOP in large letters, or snapping a rubber band (Seligman, 1991). Once the thoughts are momentarily interrupted attention can be shifted to something else, be it a project, activity, or object in the immediate environment. Another method is to write down the thoughts when they occur, and set a time to think about them later. It is important to make a commitment not to think about them until that time.

Disputation, or arguing against un-helpful beliefs, is a longer lasting solution than distraction. By effectively disputing the beliefs that lead to unwanted feelings and behavioral reactions, individuals can change their responses (Seligman, 1991). To dispute a thought, imagine someone else has said the negative belief to you, and then fight back. Conjure as much evidence as possible, and look for alternative explanations than those held by the belief. Decatastrophize by asking yourself what the implications are, and how likely any awful implications might be. Also, look at the usefulness of holding the belief, is the belief helpful or harmful in itself? Finally, detail all of the ways that the situation can be changed for the better.

After completing ABC and D, take note of the ways that your feelings and behavioral reactions change for the better. If the disputation process is successful, people generally feel energized (Seligman, 1991). If you'd like, record the "Energization" as the E in your ABCDE process.

<u>Resilience Exercise</u>

"Men are disturbed not by things
but by the views which they take of them."
-Epictetus

"There is nothing either good or bad,
but thinking makes it so."
-Shakespeare, Hamlet

When faced with an adversity, complete the following steps:

1. Pick a recent event that elicited an emotional response and/or behavioral reaction. Bring the details of the event to mind and write down an objective account of the "who, what, when, and where." Do not include any interpretation of the event in this step.

2. Describe the automatic thoughts you had in response to this event. Write down quotes from your "internal monologue" relating to the event.

3. Describe the emotions you felt and any behavioral responses you had.

4. How are the thoughts and the emotions connected? If your thoughts about the event had been different, would your emotional and behavioral responses be different as well?

5. In the end, were your behavioral and emotional reactions helpful or harmful? If they were not helpful, make note of the beliefs connected with the harmful consequences.

6. Check the unhelpful beliefs for thinking errors and inaccuracies. If the beliefs are not accurate or fall into a habitual pattern of thought, dispute or argue against the unhelpful beliefs with all of your ability. Conjure undermining evidence and generate alternative explanations.

7. Note the difference in the way you feel. What has changed as a result of completing this process?

Conclusion

Since positive psychology was founded, a great deal of knowledge has been gained by re-directing scientific inquiry toward the positive aspects of life. However, the work has just begun. In the future, many hope to have a classification system for the characteristics of human flourishing that is just as extensive as that which we currently have describing mental illness. This handbook is intended to add to the rapidly growing body of research-based literature examining the "good life."

Through its tips and suggested interventions, this handbook also addresses the applied aspect of positive psychology. Members of the field are adamant that positive psychology be an applied discipline. Studying the "good life" is not enough; we must apply this knowledge to transform people's lives and the world. Positive psychology has been successfully applied in a surprising number of domains including education, coaching, business, military training, medicine, law, and more. Individuals can make a difference by utilizing their strengths and applying positive psychology to their unique circumstances. Through our shared work and commitment, I believe we can make Martin Seligman's goal of 51% of the world's population flourishing by 2051, a reality.

<u>**Acknowledgements**</u>

It is an honor for me to thank the people who have played a role in my personal development, and the creation of this handbook. I owe my deepest gratitude to the professors, teachers, staff, and students who contributed to my educational experience at the University of Pennsylvania's Master of Applied Positive Psychology program. You are amazing people who are changing the world, and I am continually inspired by you. I know that I am forever changed by the knowledge and relationships I gained in the MAPP program.

I would like to offer special thanks to my advisor Dan Bowling, who gives an exceptional amount of his time and energy teaching in the MAPP program, and who guided me through the process of writing and publishing this handbook.

Finally, I would like to thank my family, friends, and co-workers who support me in pursuing my dreams. To my friends and mentors from Universal Spirit Center, thank you for making my road to MAPP a success. To Margaret and Nate, thank you for helping me complete this second edition. To my coach Jane, thank you for the major role you play in my continuing growth. To Emily, my closest friend and partner in the application of positive psychology, thank you for the beautiful things we've done and will do together. To my father and brother, thank you for your love and unconditional support. And finally, to my mother, thank you for being the single largest contributor to this handbook, I could not have done it without you.

With love,

Jessica

<u>**References**</u>

Baumeister, R., Gailliot, M., DeWall, C.N., and Oaten, M. (2006). Self-regulation and personality: How interventions increase regulatory success, and how depletion moderates the effects of traits on behavior. *Journal of Personality*, 74(6), 1773-1801.

Bryant, F.B. (2003). Savoring beliefs inventory: A scale for measuring beliefs about savoring. *Journal of Mental Health*, 12(2), 175-196.

Cooperrider, D. L., Whitney, D., & Stavros, J. M. (2008). *Appreciative inquiry handbook*. (2nd ed.). Brunswick, Ohio: Crown Custom Publishing.

Coutu, D. (2002). How resilience works. *Harvard Business Review, 80*(5), 46-55.

Csikszentmihalyi, M. (2008). *Flow: The psychology of optimal experience*. New York, NY: HarperCollins Publishers.

Diener, E., & Biswas-Diener, R. (2008). *Happiness: Unlocking the mysteries of psychological wealth*. Malden, MA: Blackwell Publishing.

Feudtner, C. (2005). Hope and the prospects of healing at the end of life. *The Journal of Alternative and Complementary Medicine*, 11(1), S-23-S-30.

Feudtner, C. (2010, January 8) Hope, Emotions, and the Provision of Palliative Care. Powerpoint lecture presented in MAPP 702. University of Pennsylvania, Philadelphia, PA.

Fredrickson, B.L. (2009). *Positivity*. New York, NY: Crown Publishers.

Fredrickson, B.L., & Losada, M.F. (2005). Positive affect and the complex dynamics of human flourishing. *American Psychologist, 60*(7), 678-686.

Gable, S.L., Asher, E.R., Reis, H.T., and Impett, E.A. (2004). What do you do when things go right? The intrapersonal and interpersonal benefits of sharing positive events. *Journal of Personality and Social Psychology*, 87(2), 228-245.

Gable, S.L., Gonzaga, G.C., and Strachman, A. (2006). Will you be there for me when things go right? Supportive responses to positive event disclosures. *Journal of Personality and Social Psychology*, 91(5), 904-917.

Gailliot, M.T., and Baumeister, R.F. (2007). The physiology of willpower: Linking blood glucose to self-control. *Personality and Social Psychology Review*, 11(4), 303-327.

Giacomo, B., Emmons, R.A., and McCullough, M.E. (2004). Gratitude in practice and the practice of gratitude. In P.A. Linley and S. Joseph (Eds.) *Positive Psychology in Practice* (pp. 464-481). New Jersey: John Wiley and Sons, Inc.

Haidt, J. (2006). *The happiness hypothesis: Finding modern truth in ancient wisdom.* New York: Basic Books.

James, W. (1892/1984). *Principles of psychology: Briefer course* (pp. 125-138). Cambridge, MA: Harvard University Press.

Latham, G.P., & Locke, E.A. (2006). Enhancing the benefits and overcoming the pitfalls of goal setting. *Organizational Dynamics*, 35(4), 332-340.

Locke, E.A. (1996). Motivation through conscious goal setting. *Applied and Preventive Psychology*, 5, 117-124.

Lopez, S.J., and Louis, M.C. (2009). The Principles of strengths-based education. *Journal of College and Character*,10(4), 1-8.

Lyubomirsky, S. (2008). *The how of happiness: A scientific approach to getting the life you want*. New York, NY: The Penguin Press.

Peterson, C. (1991). The meaning and measurement of explanatory style. *Psychological Inquiry*, 2(1), 1-10.

Peterson, C. (2006). *A primer in positive psychology*. Oxford: Oxford University Press.

Peterson, C., & Seligman, M.E.P. (2004*). Character strengths and virtues: A handbook and classification*. Oxford: Oxford University Press.

Pink, D.H. (2009). *Drive: The surprising truth about what motivates us*. New York, NY: Riverhead Books.

Post, S.G. (2005). Altruism, happiness, and health: it's good to be good. *International Journal of Behavioral Medicine*, 12(2), 66-77.

Post, S., & Neimark, J. (2007). *Why good things happen to good people*. New York, NY: Broadway Books.

Rath, T., & Conchie, B. (2008). *Strengths based leadership*. New York, NY: Gallup Press.

Reivich, K. (2010, March 27) Savoring. Powerpoint lecture presented in MAPP 708. University of Pennsylvania, Philadelphia, PA.

Reivich, K., & Shatté, A. (2002). *The resilience factor*. New York, NY: Broadway Books.

Richardson, G.E. (2002). The metatheory of resilience and resiliency. *Journal of Clinical Psychology*, *58*(3), 307-321.

Schwartz, B. (2004). *The paradox of choice: Why more is less*. New York, NY: HarperCollins Publishers.

Seligman, M.E.P. (1991). *Learned optimism*. New York, NY: Alfred A. Knopf, Inc.

Seligman, M.E.P. (2002). *Authentic happiness*. New York, NY: Free Press.

Seligman, M.E.P. (Artist). (2009). *Dr. martin seligman's top strengths*. [Web]. Retrieved from
http://www.youtube.com/watch?v=YC1HZqCbZ70andNR=1

Seligman, M.E.P., & Csikszentmihalyi, M. (2000). Positive psychology: an introduction. *American Psychologist*, 55(1), 5-14.

Seligman, M. E. P. (2011). *Flourish: A visionary new understanding of happiness and well-being.* New York, NY: Free Press.

Sheldon, K. M., Kashdan, T. B., & Steger, M. F. (2011). *Designing positive psychology: Taking stock and moving forward* . New York: Oxford University Press.

Snyder, C.R. (2002). Hope theory: rainbows in the mind. *Psychological Inquiry*, 13(4), 249-275.

So, T.T.C. (2009, July 18). Well-being at the population level: building a flourishing world. *Positive Psychology News Daily*, Retrieved from http://positivepsychologynews.com/news/timothy-so/200907183566

Tice, D.M., Baumeister, R.F., Shmueli, D., and Muraven, M. (2006). Restoring the self: Positive affect helps improve self-regulation following ego depletion. *Journal of Experimental Social Psychology*, 43(3), 379-384.

Vaillant, G. (2008). *Spiritual evolution: A scientific defense of faith.* New York: Broadway Books.

Wiechman, B,M,, & Gurland, S.T. (2009). What happens during the free-choice period? Evidence of a polarizing effect of extrinsic rewards on intrinsic motivation. *Journal of Research in Personality*, 43(4), 716-719.

Whitworth, L., Kimsey-House, K., Kimsey-House, H., & Sandahl, P. (2007). Co-active coaching: New skills for coaching people toward success in work and life. (2 ed.). Boston, MA: Davies-Black.

www.ingramcontent.com/pod-product-compliance
Lightning Source LLC
Chambersburg PA
CBHW051222250726
48655CB00006B/2547